Corona Infection! The Odyssey

Where are the family doctors during the pandemic?

Inès D´Alena

Copyright © 2021 Inès D´Alena
All rights reserved and for any contact is the legal
representation in Germany:

Inès Pons y Nobis, Rothgerberbach 4, 50676 Köln

No part of this book may be translated, reproduced, or stored in a retrieval system, or transmitted in any form or
by any means, electronic, mechanical, photocopying,
recording, or otherwise, without express written
permission of the publisher.
ISBN: 9798598834893

DEDICATION

This book is dedicated to all medical staff around the world who work tirelessly to save lives.

Corona Infection! The Odyssey

CONTENTS

Introduction	09
Preface	10
January - March	13
09 – 12 March	15
13 – 15 March	21
16 – 18 March	25
19 – 22 March	34
23 – 27 March	38
28 March - October	43
November– December	49
The virus	52
Yes, We Can	57
About the author	61

Corona Infection! The Odyssey

ACKNOWLEDGMENTS

My family doctor answered all my medical questions patiently. At the beginning of the pandemic in April 2020, he treated Corona virus infected people in their homes, who will never forget his help.

My caring neighbors actively offered their help during my illness and were always at my side.

With family and friends at home and abroad I always found support - because of the distance it often only took place by phone, but was very important for me.

Thank you!

INTRODUCTION

On Wednesday, March 18, I became dizzy shortly after getting up. Much to my regret, the strong breakfast coffee was just hot and liquid, but without any taste, and between each sip came the strong cough.

Suddenly, on my right hand, between my thumb and index finger, I noticed a bruise of about 3 cm, almost round, which looked like a hematoma. I couldn't remember getting hurt...

When I tried to put on my socks, I also saw a large dark discoloration on my big toe, which certainly wasn't present the day before.

Finally, I had creamed myself after the bath and I would have noticed the strange color of my toe!

It was also impossible that I had bumped into something at night in my sleep, as I owned a large padded bed that didn´t have hard edges.

Thoughtful, coughing, tired, without taste and smell and with a slight dizziness, I made the hour-long morning walk with my pet and then called my doctor´s office…

PREFACE

I am living in Germany where I was borne and this book has been translated into different languages, because I want to share my story with many people around the world.

This book is in one part the story of my life-threatening medical history in spring 2020. At the same time, it contains a record of many events that have taken place around the world in that year.

My father was a general practitioner with his own practice, my mother was a medical and technical assistant and several other family members were also active in medical professions. A surgeon and a naturopath were among my uncles, and my aunts also worked in hospitals.

Countless family reunions took place, during which most of the talk was about medicine and of course I learned about it above average. My interest in this subject was and still is existing – to my great happiness, as it turned out during my Covid-19 illness!

When I fell ill in March 2020, no personal examinations were carried out for respiratory disease. Fearing infection with the new corona virus within the doctor's offices, patients were automatically given a Certificate of incapacity for work over seven days per mail.

This approach was based on the WHO recommendations and has been handled in this way by many countries around the world.

In my case, the medical side diagnosed an influenza infection after a telephone call. A personal examination did not take place in the later course of my illness.

I did not see myself in danger because I was physically very fit and doing sports. I spent a lot of time outdoors with my dog. I didn't have any of the pre-existing conditions that, according to the WHO and the Robert Koch Institute in Germany, could lead to problems with flu or Covid-19.

However, the way of my illness was completely different than I ever expected! No one had previously reported that an infection with the corona virus could have other consequences than a severe and life-threatening pneumonia. All the media around the world informed us viewers, listeners and readers about a possible threat of suffocation in overcrowded hospitals and no one had a cure.

My symptoms, however, did not indicate an infection with the new pathogen as described before.

At the time, after detecting my strange ailments, I kept a "list" of my symptoms, which months later turned out to be common problems with SARS-CoV2 infections. These can lead to death without early treatment!

Fortunately, I have correctly identified two particularly dangerous symptoms of a Corona virus infection during my course of the disease without even knowing it at the time! If I hadn't grown up as the daughter of a doctor, I wouldn't have noticed them and might have died overnight... as others before!

I fought them with medication, which, Thanks God, I had available at home. Similar medicines are also used in hospitals during the treatment of patients. Unfortunately, the disease has often advanced so far, that in many cases it is hardly treatable...

My life-threatening symptoms, the effects of which, together with my "self-treatment", were known to only a few people in my environment at the time. After surviving illness, at the end of March 2020, I also informed my family doctor. He listened to me very attentively and also very astonished, but could not attribute the described symptoms to any known illness.

In May 2020, I posted via Twitter how I used to fight the disease.

Since then, months have passed, my different sufferings at that time are now known worldwide as usual SARS-CoV-2 symptoms. My doctor remembers everything I told him at the time. But people of all ages on all continents are still dying because of the Corona virus!

Here is my story...

JANUARY TO MARCH

Since the confirmed appearance of the virus, many people had already died with, on and because of the virus, while the rest of the world was still relatively uninvolved at the beginning of 2020. In Germany, too, it was no different.

I live in the city of Cologne in Western Germany, work full-time in the tourism industry and thus I am in constant professional contact with people from all over the world. In January 2020, the International Furniture Fair took place in the city, which lasts for several days, and in February, as every year, the International Confectionery Fair.

Both are major events, so-called "world fairs", which attract thousands of trade fair exhibitors and visitors from all possible countries.

The Cologne hotels are then fully booked at maximum prices, the subways full of travelers from Asia, South America and Europe. The restaurants and shops make a great turnover thanks to the many tourists and businessmen. The same applies, of course, to carnival week, which began this year shortly after the fairs in February. As every year, hundreds of thousands of people came to the city, which then experienced a state of emergency for a week.

By the way, many other cities around the world also host international fairs and carnival celebrations.

While we professionals in the tourism, event and catering industries had a lot to do under normal working conditions, my colleagues and myself were surprised by an unusually high number of sick guests. Usually there is always a sick guest, but this year there were more cases of illness, some of which even had to be admitted to a hospital.

However, the people affected were usually quickly released at their own request, as they preferred to return to their home country for treatment near their family.

From a retrospective point of view, it is clear to me that everything had to come as it came. The virus had already begun its journey around the world with the help of the many travelling people!

At the beginning of the year, there were hardly any recommendations or even instructions from the government and health authorities for a better protection against the corona virus, which had already raged in China, spread further throughout Asia and was already to be found on European soil.

As always, planes took off to carry countless people around the globe, and everyone thought to be safe from infection.

Why should a tiny, invisible virus keep away humanity from living normally? So, the pandemic also gained momentum in Germany, which I could not escape.

However, the way of my illness was completely different than I ever expected!

09 TO 12 MARCH 2020

On Monday, March 9th 2020, I woke up with a frenzied headache, which intensified during the day and also resisted several Ibuprofen 400.

On the radio, the presenter announced that Italy had declared itself a restricted zone because of many SARS-CoV-2 infections and had imposed a curfew. The first German citizen had died as a result of a Corona virus infection.

The horrific bushfires in Australia were still uncontrollable. Thousands of people were affected, and millions of animals had already been burned.

In Ireland, the St. Patrick's Day parades were also cancelled nationwide.

Nevertheless, I tried to approach the working day as normal as possible, but the pain in my head made the day hell for me. I struggled to focus on simple routine tasks.

Every time the phone rang on my desk, a kind of lightning pain passed through my brain.

As the evening approached, I was overjoyed to be able to go home. Completely exhausted, I wished myself a quiet, relaxing night and even let dinner fail. At 7 pm, I lay down in bed and watched a film before sleep, which actually helped me to slide into the realm of dreams.

Stupidly, I felt a very strong urge to urinate throughout the night, which made me wake up several times to walk into the bathroom.

I couldn't believe it and wondered where all the liquid I was leaving, came from!? I hadn't drunk more during the day than on other days and usually I had slept through the night.

After this unexpectedly short night's sleep, I woke up on the morning of March 10th 2020 without a hint of headache, but the first sneezing after getting up was just the beginning of a series of over a hundred episodes that lasted all over the day.

Since I had a single office, my colleagues didn't have to worry about contagion and I just kept working as normal as possible. The urge to urinate was as strong as the night before, and I briefly thought of a cystitis.

Around noon, my eyes began to itch, and in the mirror, I noticed a strong redness of my conjunctiva. Obviously a cold was waiting for me, but I didn't see the need for a doctor's visit.

The following Tuesday, March 11. 2020 brought a new surprise - no more sneezing, even the strong urge to urinate had completely disappeared.

Instead, I had sore throats that made me think of tonsillitis in its intensity! Even my ears were affected and hurt by every touch.

The telephone receiver on my eavesdroppers was hard to bear. Fortunately, my eyes had lost their redness and did no longer hurt.

I wondered about the changing clinical picture, but I wasn't worried about it, because I wasn't worse off, but only differently every day and mastered my working day with flying colors. All my colleagues kept their distance from my office and I from them as well as from the customers.

During the day, I learned over the radio that the WHO had declared a global pandemic because of the spread of SARS-CoV-2, as many countries had reported more and more infected and deaths.

As I lay down to sleep that evening, I secretly wondered what to expect after my awake.

The first thing that happened on March 12. 2020, right after getting up, was unexpected.

A terrible coughing fit struck me, and shook me right through. Even a quarter of an hour later, I was not able to brush my teeth without leaving away the toothbrush several times, because the coughing stimulus was simply too strong. However, miraculously all other complaints had disappeared!

While drinking my first coffee of the day, I pondered the daily changing ailments: headaches, sneezing, urinary urges, sore throats, eye and ear pain and cough...

But as the complaints changed daily and did not occur together, I decided to just continue my professional activity.

This time, however, I had real difficulty doing any work, because even the simple telephone service was no longer possible because of the coughing fits, which became more and more violent in the course of the morning.

The owner of the company called me during the morning and after a few sentences she changed with me, she decided to send me home or to the doctor immediately. She feared that I might have contracted the flu and did not want to lose any more staff because of an illness, otherwise she would have had to step in herself because of a lack of staff.

I did not protest, packed up my belongings and said goodbye to my colleagues, who wished me well.

Shortly before the closure of my GP practice, I made it to the reception where the staff member urged me to go home immediately to call the doctor from there and not to return to the medical cabinet as long as I was ill.

I was very surprised because my father had been a doctor with his own medical office. Throughout my life, I had only experienced that doctors take care of the sick personally and on "sight" because the medical history must be before diagnosis.

On that day, however, everything went differently...

I was really astonished and coughing, when my GP shortly afterwards on the phone explained that the procedure of his practice was based on the recommendations of the Robert Koch Institute (RKI). This is the sanitary center of disease in Germany.

Currently, only simple telephone "examinations" in patients with respiratory diseases should take place. A certificate of incapacity for work should be sent by mail in order to avoid possible infections by the corona virus within the practice. There were also some specially worked-out questions that I had to answer. The answers should help to find out a possible infection with SARS-CoV-2.

The questions were:

1) Have you recently been to a risk area?
2) Did you have contact with an infected person?
3) Do you have a fever?

I truthfully answered negatively all three questions, but as a hotel clerk with constant public traffic, I still told my GP that many people from high-risk areas were close to me. The Cologne subway was also packed with people from all sorts of countries!

And how should I know if there was not an infected person among them who did not know it himself? In addition, I did not have a fever since my childhood, but at most increased temperature.

Since I had to cough several times during the phone call, the doctor, who is also a pulmonary specialist, realized that it was a productive cough that plagued me.

However, the typical corona cough was described as dry. So, it did not fit well as the denial of the questions, to the clinical picture of those infected with SARS- CoV-2.

When I still proposed a PCR-test, he told me that he wouldn't have one. There would be a global shortage and at the moment no objective reason for testing. He would attribute the symptoms to a flu-like infection and I would receive a seven-day certificate of incapacity for work by mail. I should get a cough juice in the pharmacy and just call again in case of deterioration.

I wouldn't have to worry about any, because according to the health office in Cologne, there were only about 60 people infected with the Corona virus.

Basically, I agreed with him, as I had also read this in the newspaper and so he ended the telephone conversation with heartfelt wishes for recovery.

After, I took my lovely big dog on a leash and we took a walk to the nearest pharmacy where I bought the recommended cough juice. On the way home, I thought about how to spend the next few days. Would the annoying cough that plagues me be replaced by something else? Or maybe something new was added?

In the evening I surfed the internet and after some reading, I ordered the first breathing masks of my life! Although I obviously only had a flu-like infection at the moment, I didn't want to risk a super infection either. After all, the new Corona virus was also among us. If the body has to fight two pathogens at the same time, this can quickly lead to overload.

I ordered them directly in China, because the Asian way to contain the pandemic seemed to me to be the right one and there were interesting specimens there. These were Nano-silver masks whose special feature is to kill bacteria and viruses through a special coating with silver particles.

The specified protection factor was 94%. The price of the masks was acceptable with 3,00 € / piece, especially as they could be washed 30 times before the silver particles lost their effect.

In addition, I decided to withdraw from everything until my recovery and only go to the fresh air with my dog. After a last sip of cough juice, I spent a very restless night.

13 TO 15 MARCH 2020

The next morning, I felt like I was wheeled, because I often woke up at night because of the strong cough and this one continued to accompany me even after getting up.

But otherwise, apart from a slight headache, I was fine.

The news informed of the closures of kindergartens and schools throughout Germany.

After the first morning walk with my dog, I went to the nearest supermarket to stock up on food for the next two weeks. It was Friday, March 13, and the business was pretty crowded.

I chose especially lots of fruits and vegetables with high vitamin C content because of health. Chocolate, marzipan and chips for the feel-good factor as well as grain bread, cheese and organic eggs.

I decided to cook with a Chinese touch and bought coconut milk, extra sharp chilly- spice as well as soy sprouts and mushrooms.

The queue of waiting people at the checkout was long and I had enough time to plan mentally the following days.

I was very happy that I had a completely free nose, could breathe well and had no other new discomfort and started looking forward to a week off at home.

I spent most of the day in front of the TV, only interrupted by two short walks with my faithful four-legged friend. Also, the night went relatively trouble-free, as the cough juice had an effect.

The following weekend of March 14th and 15th was quiet, without further surprise about new complaints. All I had left was the cough that had become stronger, but otherwise I spent time with my dog outdoors on both days.

It was very cold, but sunny, there was hardly any wind and I wanted to refuel vitamin D. When I was child, my father had taught me how important the sun vitamin is for health.

He had always insisted on going to the fresh air as much as possible, even in case of illness, and to ventilate a lot at home in order to get all the viruses/bacteria emitted during sneezing and coughing out of the house. In my apartment, all the windows were tilted, so there was a constant exchange of air and this also benefited my still existing headaches.

A state of emergency was declared in Spain on 14th of March and in France only systemically important companies such as supermarkets, banks and pharmacies were allowed to remain open.

I spoke on the phone with my family in Spain on both days to find out about the serious situation there, which was getting worse and worse.

After, I also spoke to my friends in France, where I had lived for many years to inquire about their well-being. Independently of each other, they found my cough horrible and told me about the chaotic conditions in the respective country.

Every day, there were more deaths, all of which were caused by SARS-CoV-2, and still no one understood exactly what caused the virus in the human body.

The hospitals were totally overcrowded and the infected people died partly overnight, for no apparent reason.

Everyone I spoke to had "barricaded themselves" at home and left the apartment only for shopping.

I was shocked, especially since my Italian neighbor had only bad things to tell too from her country. The scenes of the trucks full of the dead spread through television, but my personal relationship with her increased the effect of these images many times over.

On Sunday lunchtime, 15th in March, I decided to pre-cook for the next few days, so that if necessary, I would only have to take the already finished portions out of the freezer and heat them.

Cooked noodles, a vegetable mixture came into a deep large pan and were poured with coconut milk. As spices I took salt and the "extra-sharp chilly" and let everything simmer together for 20 minutes. In between, I tasted it and added chilly several times, as its taste was barely noticeable.

I was very annoyed about my purchase because I had imagined something different under "Chilly-extra sharp". After almost half of the spice pack had been consumed, I finally found the dish delicious, then ate part of it as a lunch meal and froze the rest.

Afterwards I cleaned up my apartment more badly than right, before I walked out with my dog in the March sun.
Although I felt weaker than usual, my condition, apart from the cough and the slight headache, was as usual.

The newsreader at the radio recalled that Australia had cancelled the Formula One World Championship.

In Austria, Parliament decided also on a curfew and a ban on assembly. The majority of all commercial and service enterprises had to close.

16 TO 18 MARCH 2020

The first coffee of the day has always been very important to me. I love him beautifully strong with a dash of milk and along with a dose of nicotine from my e-cigarette.

On this Monday morning, March 16th 2020, I had to reinforce the freshly brewed filter coffee in my cup with 2 heaped spoons of instant coffee to taste anything at all. But there was an additional taste that was indefinable.

Somehow strange, unknown, metallic...

Coughing, I cooked two 7-minute organic eggs, and when I ate them with salt on a bun for breakfast, the same thing happened as before – it tasted nothing and there was only a strange, slight metallic taste left in my mouth!

After this strange experience, which really has absolutely no similarities with the "paper taste" of food in case of a flu or a flu-like infection, I was at first perplexed. In addition, there was obviously a loss of my sense of smell.

Although my nose was absolutely free, the sense of smell didn't seem to work, as I hadn't noticed the smell of brewing my filter coffee. Normally, the beloved coffee smell moved through my apartment, but today it was missing - what was that??

I decided to continue to observe these symptoms, but since they didn't hurt or seemed to be anything bad at first glance, it didn't seem dangerous to me either.

Luckily, I couldn't find a problem with my lungs, my breathing was normal and my 25,00 € expensive pulse oximeter confirmed to me an oxygen content of

99% in my blood. So, first everything seemed to be OK!

The news of Radio Cologne reported of company closures throughout Germany, which were intended to curb the spread of the Corona virus. The affected employees either continued to work in the home office or were sent to short-time work.

Most daycare centers and all schools had been yet closed for several days and all major events, fairs and other events had been cancelled.

The number of people infected increased daily and there was a debate at government level about drastic measures to combat the new Corona virus definitively, until the Federal Government announced to the citizens an imminent shutdown in Germany starting on March 23th 2020.

Several European countries had already sealed off their borders to all travelers in order to better control what was happening in their country.

Traffic jams of round about 100 km formed before the borders, as the trucks with deliveries of all kinds were not excluded.

The United States of America had already isolated itself from the rest of the world, as had Australia, New Zealand, and Asia, in view of the daily increase in the number of infected peoples there.

On the African continent, the south was particularly affected by the Corona virus.

For the first time in modern history, congregations of believers were no longer allowed in all churches, mosques and synagogues.

After a sunny, fresh day, when the air in the city seemed clear and pure like never before, I prepared a portion of my frozen meal for dinner. A few forks of it were enough to remind me the extent of my loss of taste.

Despite a lot of spice "Chilly-extra- sharp" I could not taste anything and only the consistency of the different ingredients made a difference between my teeth. I ate my whole plate, but only because I felt a weak feeling in my stomach.

I was interpreting it as hunger and after that I went to sleep early.

The stomach pains that occurred at night, awakened me and were the harbinger of a severe diarrhea that lasted the whole day of March 17th.

Forcibly, I spent most of the day at home, taking a tablet against diarrhea and additionally taking another one to combat stomach pain. Maybe my pains came from too much sharp- Chilly, whose taste I couldn't even perceive?

By evening, the diarrhea was over, as was the pain in my stomach. Only the cough, like the loss of smell and taste, persisted. I felt quite groggy and after a full bath with a lot of foam, I went to sleep early.

My dog came to me conspicuously often during this time, because he felt exactly that I was not doing very well and was content with several short runs outside.

On Wednesday, March 18, I became dizzy shortly after getting up. Much to my regret, the strong breakfast coffee was just hot and liquid, but without any taste, and between each sip came the strong cough.

Suddenly, on my right hand, between my thumb and index finger, I noticed a bruise of about 3 cm, almost round, which looked like a hematoma. I couldn't remember getting hurt... When I tried to put on my socks, I also saw a large dark discoloration on my big toe, which certainly wasn't present the day before.

Finally, I had creamed myself after the bath and I would have noticed the strange color of my toe!

It was also impossible that I had bumped into something at night in my sleep, as I owned a large padded bed that didn´t have hard edges. Thoughtful, coughing, tired, without taste and smell and with a slight dizziness, I made the hour-long morning walk with my pet and then called my doctor´s office.

However, he was not present and so I was connected to his medical representative. I described my symptoms in the last few days and asked for a new certificate of incapacity for work and a personal examination.

The doctor did not see any imminent danger to me in my symptoms, but of course, I would be free to go to a hospital. A personal visit to the medical would by no means possible!

Somehow frustrated, I put the phone on and felt left alone. I didn't see any reason to stay in a hospital where a lot of people were dying, but I couldn't find my condition normal.

After, I phoned friends and family again in Germany and abroad until noon.

Suddenly, I saw that several large, itchy quads had formed on my right forearm. This picture of illness was well known to me, but it had nothing to look for on this very cool March day!

Since my youth, I have suffered from a very rare allergy called heat and pressure urticaria, which only appears when there is too much heat / pressure.

An allergy is always a sign of an excessive immune system that reacts too strongly to certain substances or stimuli that are completely banal. Many severe allergies, including mine, are often treated with cortisone as it "shuts down" the immune system and fights inflammation.

Lighter cases are often treated with an antihistamine.

Now I was really alarmed, especially since it seemed that the "blue spot" on my right hand had increased during the morning. I grabbed a stamp magnifying glass and looked at the "hematoma" that had appeared overnight for no apparent reason, as well as its counterpart on my toe. Suddenly a thought passed me through, which made me shudder!

To check my bad inkling, I spiked into a finger with a heated sewing needle and the drop of blood which came out, had the consistency of syrup. Now I was quite sure...

I definitely had a serios problem with my blood clotting, which was usually always within the norm range and was obviously in the high range at the moment!

Fortunately, as a doctor's daughter, I knew about the deadly danger of blood clots, which could, among other things, trigger thrombosis and embolism, resulting in a heart attack or stroke. Suddenly and without prior notice!

Immediately, I ran to the bathroom where I keep my medication, swallowed three tablets of aspirin 500mg, which as a thinner of my blood were supposed to dissolve the clots. Aspirin is not only a painkiller, but also a blood thinner.

I also decided to treat my rapidly spreading urticaria with a dose of 5mg prednisone, a cortisone preparation.

Basically, one should NOT suppress the immune system during a disease, as it should and must form antibodies against the existing pathogen, but to me it seemed the only right thing to do.

I had been ill for nine days since the first symptoms appeared and there had been no improvement, but only strange new symptoms had appeared. Antibodies, against whatever, should have formed a long time ago.

Obviously, my immune system was confronted with "something" that overstretched it.

Otherwise, my rare allergy would not have broken out and so I sat down in front of my laptop to record all the symptoms that occurred from the first day of my illness.

> Day 1: Very strong headaches and urge to urinate
> Day 2: Continuous urge to urinate and continuous sneezing
> Day 3: Severe sore throat, earache, aching red eyes
> Day 4: Severe cough, mild headache
> Day 5: Severe cough, headache
> Day 6: Severe cough, headache
> Day 7: Severe cough, headache
> Day 8: Severe cough, headache, stomach pain, loss of sense of smell and taste

> Day 9: Severe cough, headache, loss of sense of smell and taste, diarrhea
> Day 10: Severe cough, headache, loss of sense of smell and taste, dizziness, "hematoma / blood clots", Urticaria

The complete loss of sense of smell and taste and the formation of "hematomas / blood clots" were not comparable to any other disease that I was aware of.

Along with the apparent immune disorder, the symptoms did not fit an infection with the new corona virus also, as described so far.

Even on the Internet, after hours of research, I couldn't find any information about it, so I decided to continue my own treatment based on an immune disorder with blood clots.

Those two symptoms could become really dangerous for my life!

To promote the thinning of my blood, I drank 1 liter of water within 5 minutes.

Afterwards, I went for two hours for a walk in the green parc, which delighted my four-legged friend and exhausted me completely.

But exercise is better than lying still when blood clots are present.

After our return it was almost 5 p.m. and I had hardly eaten anything before. However, I wasn't hungry and I couldn't taste anything anyway. I inspected the "hematoma" on my hand again by magnifying glass and found that it had not spread any further.

The border, which I had painted with a ballpoint pen after its discovery, still fit. The urticaria on the arm had shrunk and so at least the cortisone struck.

With mixed feelings, I smeared a cheese sandwich to prepare my stomach for the coming aspirin tablets and cortisone.

As in the days before, only the consistency of my dinner was recognizable. No taste at all! In terms of taste, it could just as well have been tree bark!

That evening, I took 1000mg of aspirin and 5mg of prednisone before preparing me for a night without sleep.

In view of the blood clots, it seemed important to me to stay awake. So, I could call an emergency doctor immediately in case of a possible nightly deterioration.

I sat down in the living room, where I took the evening dose of my cough juice, which at least brought me some relief. Then I spent the time until 2 a.m. searching the Internet for reports of similar corona symptoms or histories, scouring the news from other countries.

I was stunned to read about the postponement of the European Football Championship until the summer of 2021, the huge return of the German Foreign Office of around 160,000 holidaymakers from all over the world, the entry ban imposed by the EU and very strict controls at the EU's external borders.

Italy was the country with the highest death rates to date and, like Spain and France, had already imposed a strict shutdown and something similar would probably not pass by Germany.

An almost complete shutdown of the economy coupled with a "quarantine at home" for anyone who did not have to leave their home for compelling reasons was the standard of shutdown in these countries.

Home office became the new norm whenever possible, as well as a largely low-contact life in order to infect no other person as possible.

From countries severely affected by the Corona virus, very ill Covid-19 patients were brought to Germany by plane, because they had no chance of survival in their home country due to a lack of intensive care places on site.

Around 2:00 in the morning, I looked at my right hand and the "hematoma" seemed to have become paler.

The same picture offered my toe and the urticaria was about to disappear slowly. I took a deep breath and hoped for improvement.

To stay awake, I made myself a coffee that, as usual in the last few days, had no flavor snots, but with its caffeine content achieved the desired effect. Armed with my e-cigarette, I turned back to the Internet and read all the finds able articles about SARS-CoV-2 until the early hours of March 19th 2020.

19 TO 22 MARCH 2020

After a waking up night, I took another two tablets of aspirin 500mg and one tablet of Prednisone 5mg at 6am in the morning, before going into the park in the dark with my fur nose.

This is located on the opposite side of the street of my apartment, is small and sometimes overcrowded, but very practical for me as a dog owner.

From my apartment, I have a beautiful green view from every window, which makes me forget the cologne city center. Luckily, I didn't meet any other people at this early time, and could watch a great sunrise with pink clouds while I was sitting on a bench. I dedicate myself to my dog, who happily romped across the meadow.

Since I had no appetite, let alone hunger, I ate nothing except two hard-boiled eggs during the day, but in the evening, I took again one tablet of aspirin 500 mg and one of prednisone 5mg. I had to shut down the dosage because in the meantime, a clear dissolution of the "hematomas" had taken place.

For me, it was the proof that the "blue spots" were blood clots.

Although I still recognized the "hematoma" on my hand and big toe, the success of my own treatment was unmistakable.

However, my clotting should not be overridden, because this could lead to other problems in the event of a possible accident with blood loss. It could be difficult to stop bleeding. Only a normalization of my blood clotting was planned.

Of course, thanks to the high-dose aspirin, the headaches had also disappeared, the agonizingly itchy urticaria also said goodbye and I cheered the cortisone, which had combated the obvious inflammation.

Calmly, I said goodbye to the day and started the evening with a fantasy movie to relax before falling asleep.

Friday, March 20th was the calendrical beginning of spring in 2020 and right after getting up, I learned to appreciate the absence of my sense of smell. I had slept so deeply after the woken- up night, that I had not noticed his efforts to wake me up.

He usually contacted me when he had to go outside for its needs, but this time, he had distributed the feces throughout the apartment. Apparently, nothing more was left in his intestines. He didn't want to go outside either, when I quickly put on the coat and opened the apartment door.

So, I turned on the radio, grabbed a bucket and scrubber listening to music and started a cleaning operation. As a long-time owner of various pets, I had an insensitive and easy-to-clean floor in my apartment, which made the cleaning work easy for me.

But the really impressive thing was, that I smelled absolutely NOTHING, although the amount of his legacies was immense!

The fact that such a total loss of my sense was possible, all overwhelmed me!

Until now, I had not really noticed the absence of my olfactory ability, but was only pleased about the fresh, pure air in Cologne and missed the beloved coffee smell. What struck me, was the lack of the sense of taste, which I noticed negatively every day.

Added to this subliminally permanent, strange metal taste, which persisted despite minutes of brushing teeth.

While I was getting my two-rooms-apartment clean, my thoughts were about the lack of sense of smell. In the past few days, I had noticed again and again in amazement how pure "smelled" our inner-city air without exhaust gases and found this condition really great.

And in my current situation, it was not only conducive, but thankful that I could not perceive the smell of his feces! The only question I asked myself was: How long will this total loss of my olfactory ability last?

The lack of taste was definitely more important to me and I wished it back as soon as possible - neither to taste food nor drink, is really no fun! Where was the enjoyment? I couldn't find anything positive in it...

After I finished cleaning, I approved a coffee that tasted like nothing as usual, but I still felt the effect of the caffeine.

Now, I did realize that my right hand looked completely normal, no trace of the "blood clot / hematoma". The same thing also affected my toe, which of course, I immediately examined in detail.

However, I didn't want to stop my own treatment and prescribed myself 500mg of Aspirin and one dose of prednisone 5mg for the day, as not to risk a setback.

Overall, I felt much better than the previous days, which unfortunately did not apply to my four-legged friend, who spent most of the day on his dog bed, as tired as I had been.

Only in the evening, he got better and in the course of a walk in the twilight, I collected two feces bags with at least semi-solid feces.

Those, too, were completely odorless…

My long-time companion even wanted to play and I was very happy about improving his general condition.

March 21th 2020 did not bring any new symptoms or an improvement in my cough, but overall, I felt fitter and more enterprising.

The same was true for my dog and so we spent again some time away from other people in the fresh air and let ourselves be seen by the sun.

Aspirin and cortisone continued to be my treatment method and the effect on my general condition was remarkable.

The weekend, I repeated the daily low dose of the two drugs and looked more closely at the impending shutdown of Germany, which was unique in history.

Most countries in the world were more or less in the same situation and for days there has hardly been any international flight operation. It had become noticeably quieter in the city of Cologne.

On Sunday, March 22th, the federal government announced a ban on contact to help contain the pandemic. All collections of more than two people from different households were banned from now on and could be subject to drastic penalties of up to €25,000 for infringements or quarantine violations.

The catalogue of fines launched in the following days was to be enforced by the police and the police.

23 to 27 March 2020

When the shutdown officially began on Monday, March 23th 2020, I was still on the road to recovery and woke up in the morning without a coughing fit.

I still had the cough, but to a tolerable extent. I didn't smell the filter coffee yet, and unfortunately, I still didn't taste the beloved watchmaker.

But that didn't scare me - I'd gotten used to it in the meantime.

I decided to spend the day looking at the city of Cologne in a state of emergency of shutdown and after the obligatory walking round, I sat down with my companion in the car.

It was around 10 o'clock in the morning and there were hardly any cars on the streets of Cologne despite the rush hour. All the main roads of the city as well as the bridges were swept away like empty.

On the right bank of the Rhine, the same picture appeared on all the big axes and even the parks were deserted, as far as I could judge from my car. So, city was usually only experienced on New Year's morning!

Apparently, most people had responded to the federal government's appeals.

Every citizen was urged to leave his or her apartment only for urgent errands and to maintain as little contact as possible.

Home office, homeschooling and short-time working became the new standard in Germany, as only "systemically important" institutions and shops remained open.

Long queues formed in front of the supermarkets because only a certain number of people were allowed to shop at the same time, so that the prescribed minimum distance of 1.5m could be respected.

People wearing masks were barely visible, as masks were reserved for medical staff. There was a worldwide shortage of protective equipment of all kinds.

I was very happy that I was cared for the next week and did not have to mingle with the people.

In addition, in many supermarkets, the shelves were swept away like empty: no flour or yeast, neither milk nor sugar, hardly any pasta and rice.

Even canned dishes, frozen products, hygiene items such as soap, disinfectant and hair shampoo were sold out.

The toilet paper manufacturers recorded probably the highest sales in their company history!

On March 24th and March 25th, I spent again time in my car to drive through the city to photograph the empty streets and squares.

I was walking my dog in the green and the water in the Rhine, which is the largest river in Europe, seemed to me to be as blue and clear as never!

Perhaps because of the discontinued shipping?

The chirping of the birds could be heard much more clearly than before the shutdown, as no noisy traffic drowned them out.

I rarely met other walkers and if so, it was other dog owners. I found the prevailing calm and the purity of the air fantastic.

As I was much better in terms of health, I began to

enjoy my "unemployed" life. Like millions of citizens who were on short-time work, for the first time, I had the possibility to take care of my personal concerns. I was skyping with friends to see them, did a deep cleaning of my car and decorated my apartment.

I found the time to read a book and decided to write one myself on the occasion.

Most of the illness-related symptoms had disappeared, only the cough and the loss of the sense of smell and taste remained unchanged.

Meanwhile, Japan canceled the 2020 Olympics and postponed it until the summer of 2021.

In the United States, the Senate approved a trillion-dollar stimulus package, and the German government promised economic aid to companies, self-employed and short-time workers, which totaled around 160 billion euros.

For the first time, in Spain there were more Corona deaths than in China and in India a quarantine violation was punished with 2 years in prison.

In England, the infection of Prince Charles, who went into quarantine, became known.

Prime Minister Boris Johnson also hit the virus - until that day, the government had not yet issued any special safeguards, but that was to change after the Prime Minister's illness. He spent several days in intensive care fighting with death, before introducing intrusive protective measures for the country immediately after his recovery.

In Germany, too, more SARS-CoV-2 infections occurred daily and, tragically, more and more people died.

On Friday, March 27, 2020, I happened to meet my GP, who was waiting in front of a bakery for admission. I was happy to see him and told him about my amazing illness and her strange ailments.

He looked at me with big eyes when he heard about the total loss of my sense of smell and taste. Calmly, he explained to me that these two symptoms were in the meantime considered as a significant indication of infection with the corona virus.

I was speechless before I let go of a little cheering. I had apparently had this disease and defeated it... but many unanswered questions remained!

Why didn't I got a pneumonia, which was supposed to be the main feature of Covid-19?

And what about the other problems I'd had over the last 14 days?

Were they also known as a sign of an infection with SARS-CoV-2?

I described exactly how I had identified the blood clots and treated them with aspirin.

I did the same with regard to my treatment with cortisone, which I had taken because of my obviously exuberant immune system.

My doctor could not classify these two "problems" as known Covid-19 symptoms. He assured me that he had not read about them in the medical literature or heard of them in exchange with colleagues.

The deep inner certainty that spread within me at that moment was that my observations would explain the entire course of the often fatal Sars-Cov-2 infection. I urged my doctor not to forget what I told him!

If he had other patients with similar ailments, a blood thinner would be the first approach to treatment to avoid life-threatening thrombosis and embolism in patients.

I was sure that the corona virus attacks the immune system in some way or even ensures that it does more harm than good to those affected.

My course of the disease also led to thinking of an infestation of the brain and the central nervous system with the virus. The disease not affected only the lungs, but also other organs!

My kidneys had excreted an extremely high amount of fluid at the beginning of the disease, which was completely abnormal for my conditions.

Was it just luck that my lung function had not been restricted, or did I perhaps owe my life to the high-dose aspirin and cortisone? Maybe the virus caused the same problems in countless people worldwide!?

To be sure that he understood correctly, I repeated my idea emphatically. He was astonished about my report, which he should not forget in the future.

We said goodbye very thoughtfully and full of new impressions.

28 MARCH TO OCTOBER 2020

Towards the end of the month of March, I felt healthy again, except for the remaining cough, and my sense of smell was back again as well as the sense of taste!

At the beginning of April, I had to learn about two deaths in my circle of acquaintances, as well as a very serious course of illness in a small four-year-old boy.

In April, hospitals were cordoned off like a fortress and visits to the sick were forbidden. The child has had to spend several weeks alone in a hospital, which is a terrible experience at this age. His initial discomfort did not indicate an infection with SARS-CoV-2.

Only one test brought certainty, but his course of the disease was quite different from that was usually the case in adults. It began with stomach pain, vomiting and diarrhea. In the further course of his illness, other problems were added, in which the doctors saw a similarity to a disease called "Kawasaki Syndrome".

He has bravely survived the lonely time of his treatment and has fully recovered.

Since then, these complaints have been observed more frequently worldwide in children who have tested positive for the virus.

The two deceased were, on the one hand, a 60-year-old neighbor who had always been officially healthy. He was tested positive for the virus, but had no conspicuous symptoms at the time and was placed under domestic quarantine to cure himself. A few days later, and still relatively easily ill, his relatives found him in his bed in the morning – he had died overnight.

The other deceased was a doctor himself, and I knew him for 25 years. He had a mild cold, which he himself had classified as such. Only a small cold with a slight cough, otherwise he did not feel any other discomfort for several days, as I was told.

He, too, was suddenly and completely unexpectedly taken out of his life overnight.

It happened the same to other people– in the US state of New York, around 12,000 people died from the new corona virus by the end of April 2020. The images of the ghost town of New York City appeared in all the

news and were reminiscent of a horror movie.

The hospitals were so congested that military hospital ships had to rush to the aid.

The car manufacturer General Motors was obliged by the War Weapons Law to produce ventilators and many well-known artists formed a fundraising gala via the Internet.

The Eifel Tower in Paris stood in an abandoned world metropolis. In France, there was a police-controlled exit barrier. Each citizen had to carry a "passport" filled in. From this it had to be very clear why and where one was moving.

In Spain, people were not allowed to leave their homes at all, except for the few who continued to work and to shop.

My 84-year-old aunt dared to leave her house after weeks of isolation, around 11 p.m. No one could be seen and she finally wanted to breathe fresh air again. The minute-long walk cost her several hundred euros...

In Italy, the capital Rome was orphaned and Pope Francis celebrated Easter Mass without believers in St. Peter's Square.

Vladimir Putin decided to "close" his country for the entire month of April, and the Soviet Union sank into complete silence, as did Lisbon/Portugal and most of South America's cities.

My doctor decided in April 2020 to treat several Covid-19 patients in person and in their homes.

His action began with a home visit by an elderly woman who felt sick and she was tested positive for the corona virus.

Dressed in a protective suit, he treated other Covid-19 patients in the following weeks, who also did not have to go to a hospital. They all survived the illness and were very grateful to him for his intervention and help.

He himself was not infected because he had taken the necessary precautions. I

In the late spring of 2020, the governments of most countries around the world created various hygiene rules and concepts that every company and private individuals had to implement, so that there would be no second wave of sick people after the end of the shutdown in Europe in the summer of 2020.

The stores introduced plexiglass separations to protect employees who worked exposed with public traffic. Visitors to restaurants, hair salons or sun studios had to leave their addresses for contact tracking.

Often there were "doormen" in front of supermarkets, who checked that everything was being kept correctly. Respiratory masks should be worn by anyone who was in closed public spaces. Since there was a worldwide shortage of medical masks, most people used simple fabric masks.

Their protective effect is nowhere near as high as is the case with FFP2 or Nano-silver masks.

In the United States, the African-American George Floyd died on May 25th during a police check.

A police officer knelt on his neck for eight minutes and the slowly suffocating man pleaded until his death to be let go because he could not breathe.

Following this incident, there were a lot of serious unrest and protests across the United States.

The images taken by video cameras went around the world.
Weeks of worldwide demonstrations against police violence and racism under the motto "Black Lives Matter" followed.

During the summer months, which were far too dry again, life in Europe gradually returned to normal, borders were opened and holidays were approved. As before, it was flown around the globe, the hotels and restaurants finally had guests again and were happy about their regained "freedom".

Many people felt safe from infection with the Corona virus, even though it killed thousands of people a day in the US and Brazil at the same time.

The deceased had to be "stored" in refrigerated trucks in front of the hospitals for days, because the funeral institutions were simply too overloaded. There were sometimes no burials, only mass graves.

The president of Brazil, Jair Bolsonaro, also fell ill with Corona, but therefore did not change his policy.

He continued to support the destruction of the Amazon rainforest, which has lost about half of its land in the last 70 years.

A catastrophic explosion took place in the port of Beirut/ Lebanon, injuring more than 6,000 and killing around 180 people.

In September, the overcrowded refugee camp "Moria" on the Greek island of Lesbos burned down and thousands of asylum seekers were suddenly homeless.

In the United States, the virus met finally President Donald Trump, who underwent a hospital treatment of 650,000 dollars and was discharged to health.

At the same time, various groups formed throughout Europe, colloquially referred to as "corona deniers", and these questioned the existence of the new Corona virus. According to some of them, the virus was transmitted over the new G5 telephone network, and others suspected a worldwide conspiracy by governments to decimate humanity.

Bill Gates, the founder of Microsoft, should also be complicit in the disaster. Through his donation of some hundred million Dollars, which was intended to advance the development of vaccines, they spread the following suspicion: It was planned to use the vaccine to chip people so that they could be remotely controlled by him and the governments.

Other groups called themselves "cross-thinkers" who saw a danger in the virus, but it was said to be so minimal that it was hardly worth mentioning. Countless demonstrations took place, some of them with thousands of participants, often with no hygiene requirements being observed.

They also endangered the police officers who had to accompany such events.

While companies in Germany and other European countries, often with high financial stakes, tried everything to minimize the risk of contagion to their customers and employees, these demonstrations were declared legally valid by the courts.

While in the USA and South America several thousand people per day still died with and because of SARS-CoV-2, most Asian countries as well as New Zealand had achieved a nearly 100% containment of the disease.

Those did not cause such high deaths, nor did the economy suffer significant damage.

Perhaps their models should be looked at more closely and, at least in part, copied?

NOVEMBER – DECEMBER

From November 2th 2020, Germany was in a "lockdown light" as the number of infections that had fallen over the summer months, did increased dramatically again.

In the United States of America, Donald Trump was voted out of office, and the new president, Joe Biden, promised a different political leadership than his predecessor.

The vaccines of BioNTech and Pfizer have made it into the U.S. regulatory review, as have Moderna and AstraZeneca.

The Chinese "dead virus" vaccine has been tested in the United Arab Emirates and has already been administered in China itself.

In Denmark and other countries, millions of minks carrying a new corona virus variant, were killed as a precaution. It was feared that this could jump on humans. The animals themselves were doing well...

A terrorist killed four people and injured many more on the open road during a rampage in Vienna/Austria. He was later identified as an IS supporter, and there were also searches of other suspects in Germany after the attack.

On December 16th 2020, a second "hard shutdown" was introduced in Germany, as the number of deaths rose daily.

Deaths amounted to around 950 people per day in the middle of the month. There were no more free intensive care beds in some cities and patients were turned away due to lack of treatment options. Medical staff have been working on the brink of exhaustion for some time.

People's general mood seemed to have gotten significantly worse than it had been a few months earlier. Several times in the last few weeks, I had personally experienced how mask deniers in a subway wagon had repeatedly coughed up other people and made fun of the mask wearers.

On one occasion, this behavior even led to a brawl, in which I myself was involved.

It ended with an arrest of the mask deniers and that day I realized how fit I had become again!

The pre-Christmas period was marked by a lack of Christmas markets and closed zoos, museums, cinemas and theatres.

Once again, a haircut was not possible and those, who wanted to buy Christmas presents, could only do so via the Internet, because the retail trade had also closed its doors.

A new, more contagious viral mutation appeared in Great Britain and all transport links were cut.

Also, in South Africa, the same variant of the SARS-CoV-2 virus appeared and caused a ban on entry.

Divine services for Christmas were celebrated on a small scale or only via the Internet. All family celebrations were completely "redesigned" by government instructions.

The fireworks on New Year's Eve were banned.

Everyone was waiting for a positive turnaround in 2021, when vaccination of the first population groups was going to start.

Can a better future be hoped for?

THE VIRUS

The first official illness and deaths related to a novel corona virus appeared in the metropolis of Wuhan in China in December 2019.

According to Chinese sources, they occurred with visitors to a market where animals of all kinds were offered for consumption.

There were, just for example, snakes and crocodiles, scale animals, marten dogs and even bats.

The city also houses a real high-security laboratory, which is called the "Institute of Virology Wuhan / Chinese Academy of Sciences". In this facility, deadly bacteria and viruses are "stored" for research purposes.

Scientists named this suddenly appeared, new virus SARS-CoV-2, and the dangerous disease it caused was called Covid-19.

At the beginning of the global pandemic, very little was known about the potentially deadly virus, which was described as triggering a lung disease. In the course of 2020, it became known that this was not the case and that, in principle, all vital organs could be affected.

Basically, the pathogen can affect people of all ages. People with pre-existing conditions or older seniors are more likely to experience a severe or fatal course.

However, many people often do not even know that they have a pre-existing condition that can become a problem.

Here is a scientific summary of what the virus does to the body and how:

It penetrates the body through the airways, through the bloodstream and "endothelial cells" it enters the organs. There it can damage or even destroy the cell layer of the existing "endothelial cells" on the inner surface of the blood and lymph vessels and **create inflammation**.

These cells can then discharge no or hardly any oxygen and nutrients into the organs. **Cardiovascular problems** and **organ failure** can occur.

Researchers have autopsied people who died of Covid-19 and found **blood clots** in the vessels of various organs. They also discovered inflammation of the inner skin of the vessel.

The endothelial cells are also involved in **controlling blood pressure, blood flow and blood clotting**.

Seniors are particularly often severely affected because, on the one hand, they have age-related pre-existing conditions.

On the other hand, they move significantly less than young people and often drink far too little, which also promotes the formation of blood clots.

Even allergies of all kinds could lead to a serious problem in the infected, as the immune system of allergy sufferers does not react 100% correctly and overreactions can trigger a life-threatening cytokine storm.

It is not necessary to wait for the patient to have to go to a hospital. Older people or people with pre-existing conditions can die! There can be serious consequential damage to every person!

Perhaps, GPs should carry out personal treatment of patients, rather than just making telephone diagnoses, sending the certificates of incapacity for work by post, and simply sending the sick into quarantine without further care? Perhaps all patients should be better informed about the impending risks of the dangerous blood clots and the possible cytokine storm?

Thrombosis and embolisms are caused by small blood particles coagulated that can trigger a heart attack or stroke. How quickly the blood assumes a dangerously high coagulation factor varies individually. Every person has his own norm values.

For some people, they are per standard higher than for others and could therefore lead to a dangerous course more quickly.

Who already knows his own norm values in order to be able to estimate his danger?

Blood pressure increases because of the thickened blood in the veins and arteries, because the heart needs to use more force to transport it through the body.

The cytokine storm is a violent overreaction of the immune system to a pathogen and can lead to inflammation throughout the body. It can occur in all sorts of diseases, not just Sars-Cov-2 infection.

Perhaps examinations should already take place in doctor's offices in order to determine blood clotting and inflammatory factors early on to prescribe appropriate medications by the family doctor?

In hospitals, heparin, a blood thinner and dexamethasone, a cortisone preparation, is widely used in Covid-19 patients. However, the disease has often advanced to the point where aid comes too late. At the beginning of the disease, as with me, aspirin would probably help just as well. There are enough drugs that dilute the blood. Aspirin is just one of them.

Cortisone is certainly not needed in every patient, but the control of CRP (inflammation levels) during the disease could provide clues to the respective inflammatory status of the patient.

Implementation would only be a matter of organization - protective suits for employees can also be available in a normal doctor's office, not only in hospitals. Special reception times for those suffering from Covid-19 could also be set up to eliminate the risk of contagion to other patients.

Research is being carried out around the world to find suitable virus inhibitors, but why are we trying to treat patients with Ebola and Malaria virus inhibitors?

These are the preparations Remdesivir and Chloroquine or Hydroxychloroquine.

The Ebola pathogen looks like a "worm" and is not transmitted through the air.

Malaria is passed on by mosquito bite and the build-up of the virus is also different.

Perhaps flu virus inhibitors should be used, since the structure of influenza viruses is very similar to that of corona viruses on the outside and both pathogens cause a respiratory disease?

Take a look at the photos of the various pathogens on the Internet – you will be amazed!

In any case, we cannot just carry on as before. It is really not enough, simply to quarantine all people and leave them to their own devices!

YES, WE CAN!

Fortunately, I am completely healthy again and have no consequential damage caused by my illness, as is the case with other people.

I smell the exhaust fumes of the cars in the air again and the morning coffee tastes great.

The dish pre-cooked during my illness with the spice "Chili- Extra Sharp" has proved to be absolutely inedible after my recovery - fiery, like a dish for dragons!

The cough remained until May 2020, and a severe fatigue led to an increased need for sleep over a few weeks.

My memory deficits during the peak phase of the disease were only noticeable to my friends and fortunately disappeared completely in May.

I only can confirm that this is a potentially fatal disease that can take a serious course overnight. My luck was to have learned a lot about medicine and medication from my father, and I was also very interested in the subject.

It was only for this reason that I was able to recognize and treat the blood clots myself. They also were clearly visible on my hand and toe, which is not necessarily the case with other people.

Blood clots can form in the deep leg veins and staying without movements increases the risk of getting them.

In my youth, I often cursed my rare allergy because it had restricted my lifestyle in hot summer months. Only cortisone could stop the urticaria forming all over the body, but this drug has side effects in long-term therapy. I have always taken it with caution and only by real needs.

Now I was more than happy that I had it at hand!

After researcher around the world has found out that SARS-CoV-2 actually causes all the symptoms (and more!) that I had myself, I know that my rare allergy actually warned me about the already beginning cytokine storm during my corona infection...

Together with the strange " hematomas " and the disappeared sense of smell and taste, they were really too conspicuous!

Who knows what would have happened if my already overreacting immune system had increased even further?!

We are all called upon and each individual is indispensable in combating the spread of the Corona virus. Unfortunately, the health system and the economy had also been put at risk by a section of the population.

These are not just organizations such as "cross-thinking" or similar worldwide, but completely normal people of all ages.

Despite all the information about the contagion pathways of the Corona virus, they have still not internalized the fact that they endanger not only themselves, but also their family, friends, work colleagues and neighbors through their behavior.

The sense of keeping distance of 1.5-2 meters, medical masks and general hygiene rules has apparently not yet been understood.

The viruses of a respiratory disease are transmitted mainly by air! So, keep your distance!

Disinfecting the hands is used to prevent possible transmission of the virus via sweat!

Asymptomatically means that there are no symptoms/complaints, but the disease is present and therefore the environment can be infected!

Either we humans all create this together by changing the way we act, by rethinking and taking more consideration, or many people will go under!

Worst case scenario will be, without rethinking and other actions: many more deaths and countless insolvencies, unsuspected number of unemployed persons, forced auctions of real estate, stock market crashes, bank failures and long-term consequences of infected persons due to illness.

Even a state can go bust, as the bailout aid for Spain, Italy, and Greece has shown. But these are just a few...

Students may not all be able to learn from home. The creators of culture will be on the precipice.

Not to mention the potential psychological problems that a part of humanity can suffer as a result of a shutdown, such as people in nursing homes or young children, who often cannot understand the meaning of the measures.

The consequences of the Corona pandemic, of the possible new shutdown and measures are not foreseeable without any other decisions than before - worldwide!

This book is available in several languages

Espagnol:	Corona ! Odisea de una infección
German:	Corona Infektion! Die Odyssee
English:	Corona Infection! The Odyssey
French:	Corona! Infection et Odyssée

ABOUT THE AUTHOR

Inès D´Alena grew up in a family with an above-average number of medical staff and has learned interesting facts about medicine on all possible occasions since childhood.

The father was a general practitioner, the mother and several close relatives also worked in medical professions.

She currently lives in a cosmopolitan city in Germany on the beautiful Rhine. Before that, she lived in the capital of France for many years. Paris is known as the "beautiful city of lights and love, but also for the imposing buildings, many of which are listed.

She speaks several languages, has got to know different cultures, met people from various political regimes and knows the principles of the great world religions.

Corona Infection! The Odyssey

www.ingramcontent.com/pod-product-compliance
Lightning Source LLC
Chambersburg PA
CBHW071121240526
45465CB00022B/747